Kid's Exercise

Get Your Body Moving!

(With The Animals)

This book is dedicated to James, Jac, and Taco.
I love them so!

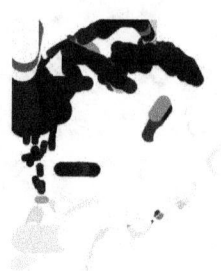

I've chosen to print the hard copy of this book in black and white to keep the price lower for the reader.
If you wish to see the art work in color, you can check out the Kindle version. Happy exercising!

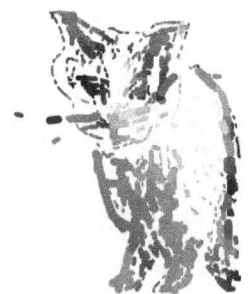

Preface

I wrote this book because I've spent the last ten summers teaching kids to get their bodies moving. And every summer I am surprised that kids are reluctant to be active and play. They really just want to watch TV or play computer games.

But we all know that!

The great thing is, I've found by the time the hour is over, in every single class, the kids are asking when I'm coming back. They've had a really fun, silly time! Kids love animals and get really creative becoming them. Just read the poems to them and watch your brilliant children act them out. They can use the movements in the book and come up with their own moves! Do these fun animal exercises with your kids and get your body moving too!

CHAPTERS

WARM UP!

Chapter 1

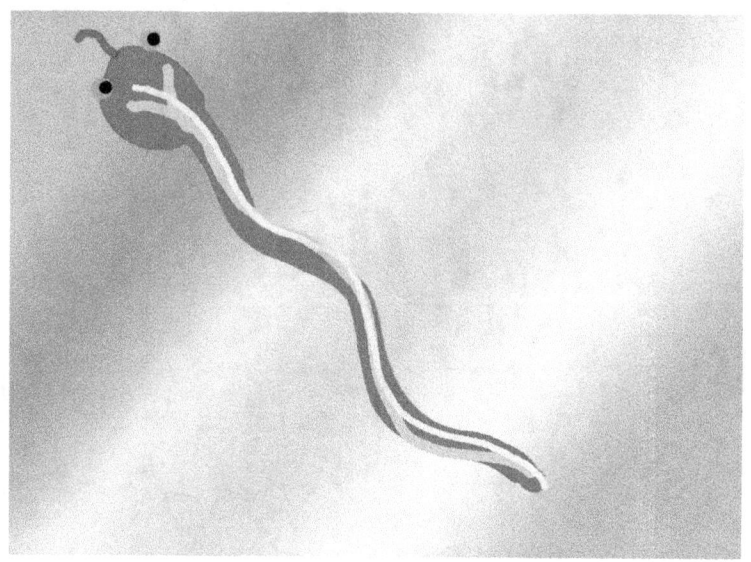

Slippery Snake

Slippery snake slithers on the floor.
Slither across the room til you can sssslither no more.
Slither up the tree, reach for the ssssun.
Now sssslither right down next to sssssomeone.
Ssssss up, sssss down.
Put a Smile on your face, now make a frown.
Slide towards the window, slide towards the door.
Now lay on the ground and slide no more.
REPEAT 3 TIMES

(After poem ask kids to name some snakes. Then have them act them out.)

Chapter 2

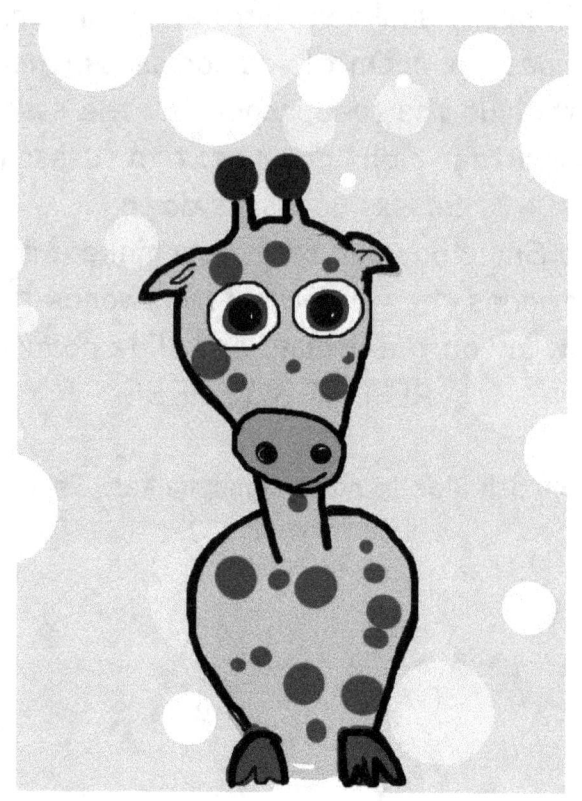

Giraffe

Stretching up his neck through trees.
Trying hard to eat some leaves.
Nips a bird perched on a twig.
Hops on one leg does a jig.
Stretch your neck up, way up high.
Then round the world, and other side.
Hungry Giraffe stands very proud.
Stands so tall to reach a cloud.

(After poem, have kids stretch their arms up, one at a time,
and side to side.)

Time
To
Move!

GET READY! LET'S GO!

Chapter 3

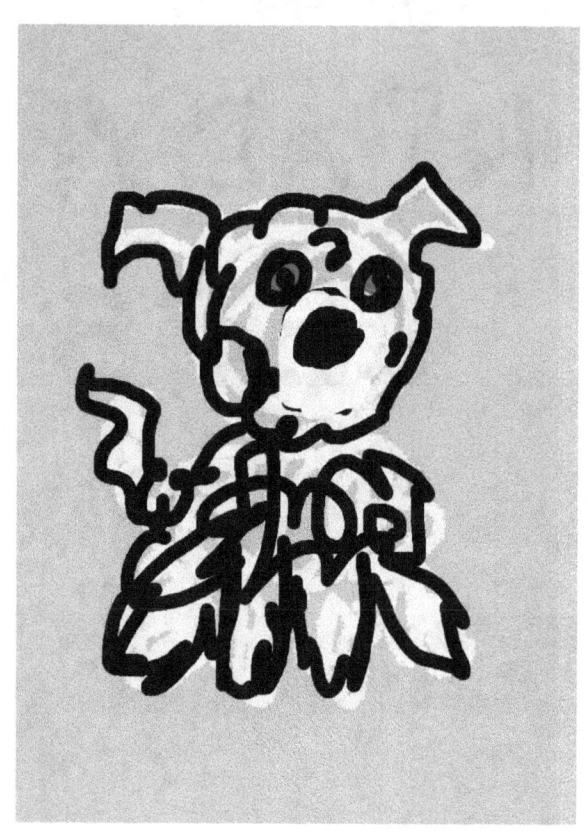

Do the wet dog

Shake your head left and right.
Shake your but with all your might.
Shake your shoulders then your feet.
Take 2 steps forward and jump and leap.
Do the wet dog! I know you can.
Do the wet dog! Now do it again.
REPEAT

(After poem, do dog training with the kids, sit, roll over....)

Chapter 4

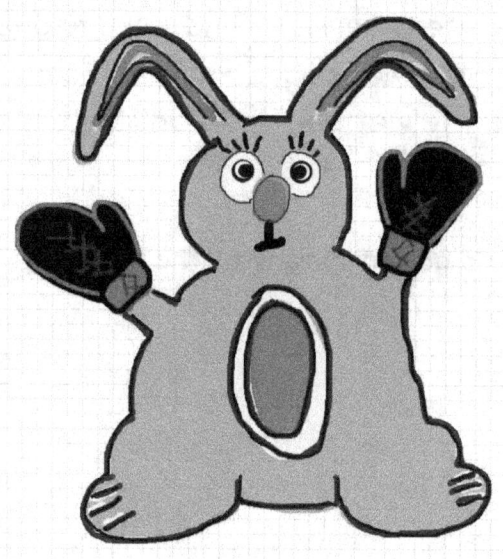

Zack Bunny Boxer

Hippity Hippity hop, Hippity Hippity hop
Hands in the air, and bop, bop, bop.
Hippity Hippity hop, Hippity Hippity hop.
Put your hands in the air and bop, bop, bop.
Go in a circle round you go.
Don't stop yet no, no, no.
Turn in a circle the other way.
Hips go back and sway, sway, sway.
Hippity Hippity hop, Hippity Hippity hop
Hands in the air, bop, bop, bop.
Hippity hippity hop, hippty hippity hop
Hands in the air bop, bop, bop.

(After poem, have kids box pretend boxers.)

Chapter 5

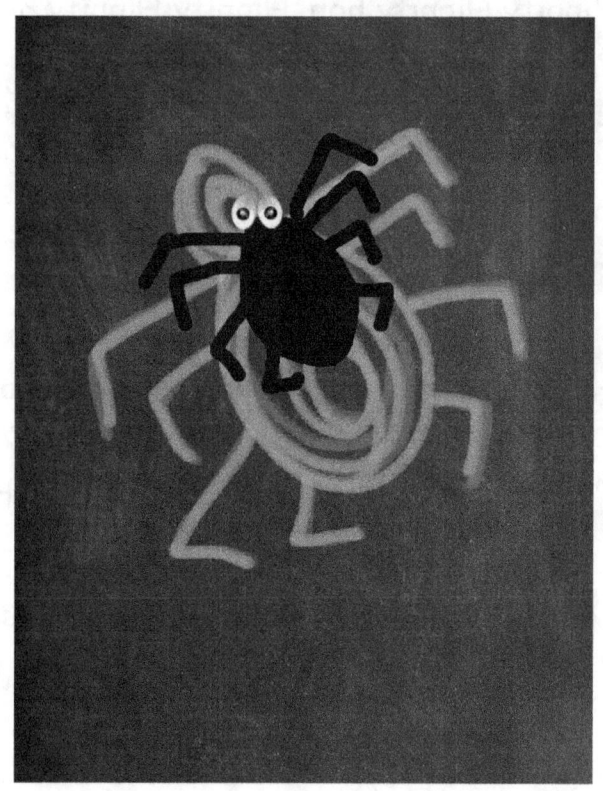

Sam the Spider

Sam the spider climbing up the wall.
Spinning a web very small.
Spinning, spinning fast as he can.
He gets too dizzy to try to stand.
He's got 8 legs shaking around.
Jumping up high, then lands on the ground.
Spinning, spinning fast there he goes.
Where he lands nobody knows.
Sam the spider finishing the web.
goes to sleep on his tiny little head.

(After poem, have the kids become a spider web shaking in the wind.)

Chapter 6

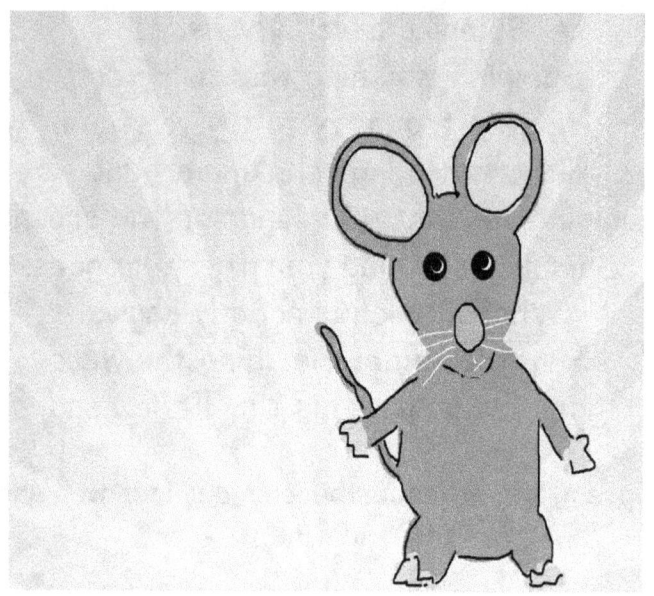

Little Mouse

Little mouse, little mouse running round the house.
Looking very small, running up the wall.
Lookin' round the room, decides to go zoom, zoom.
Special little guy, jumpin' very high.
Isn't he so cute with his little face?
Thinkin' he's a car, in a mousy race.

(After poem, do a mouse relay race.)

Chapter 7

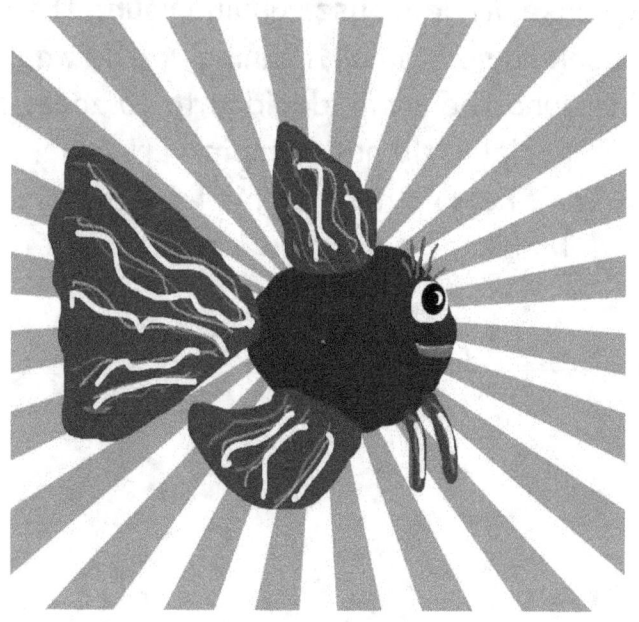

Fishfinger

Splish, Splash
There's a fish in the water and he's stuck on his back.
He looked at his bottom, and he saw his fin.
And he tried to turn over so he did it again.
He isn't a Goldfish.
He isn't a Trout.
He isn't a Blowfish with a big fat pout.
He's got big whiskers blowing bubbles out his lips.
And he's trying to turn over so he's rolling his hips.
He's a little ole Betta fish with a face kinda funny.
And he caught a big wave and finally turned on his
tummy.

(After poem, have kids roll from their backs to their
stomachs on the floor several times.)

Chapter 8

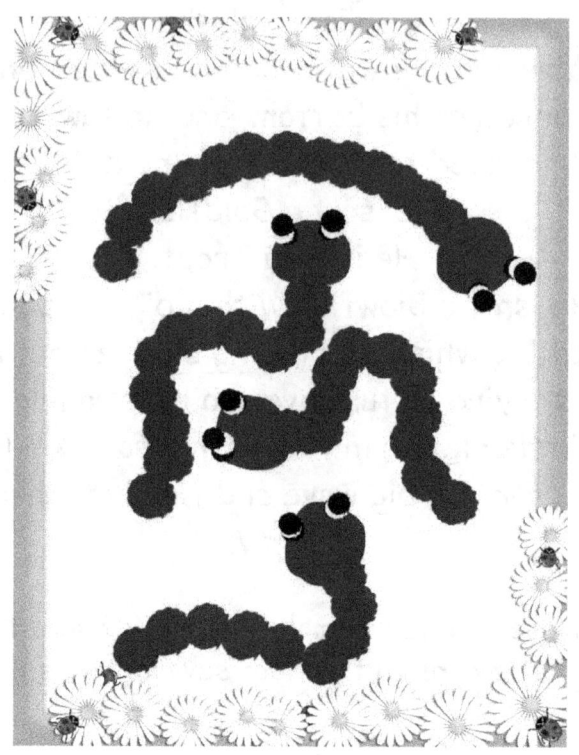

Wiggly Worm

Put your hands in the air and spread your fingers wide.
Wiggly, wiggly worms slip and slide.
Arms straight out and wiggle fingers round.
Now put them in the garden, straight into the ground.
Now climb up the fence, way up on our toes.
And wiggle those worms like nobody knows.
Now come on down with a wiggly worm stance.
And sit right down, end of wiggly worm dance.
REPEAT

(After poem; have kids clap as loud as they can, and jump as high as they can.)

Chapter 9

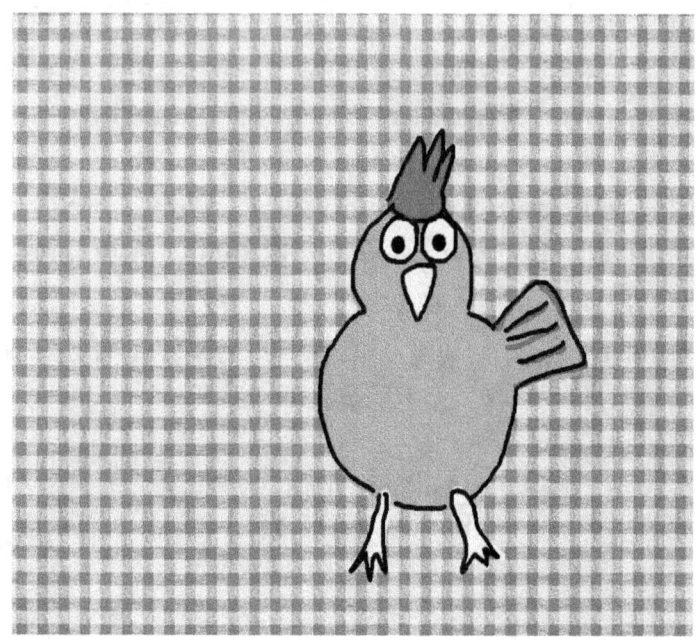

Chicken

Clucky, clucky chicken walks around the farm.
Flapping her wings 'cause she doesn't have arms.
Clucky, clucky chicken, a squawk from within.
Dancing a little dance as she sticks out her chin.
She's looking for her rooster as she dances all around.
She's looking for her rooster as she goes up and down.
Grabbing another chicken she swings on her feet.
Clucky, clucky chicken swinging to the beat.
REPEAT

(After poem do a Dosey Do with kids.)

Chapter 10

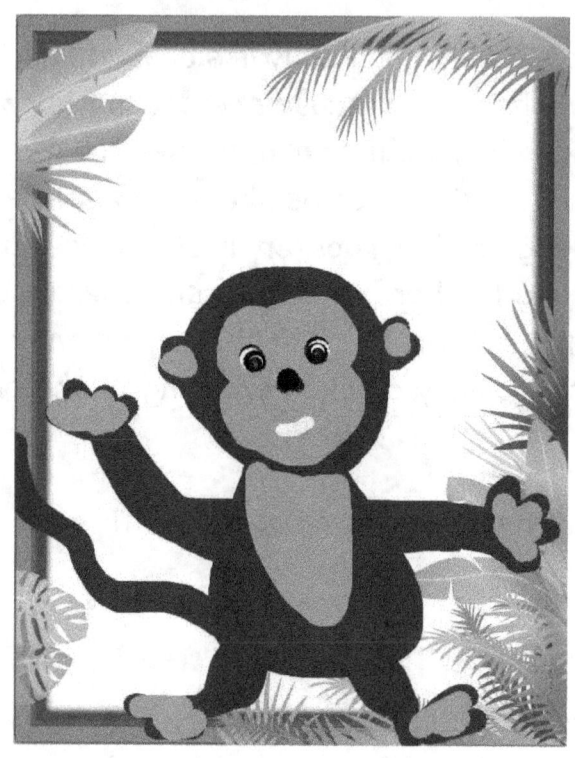

Danni Monkey

Come on you monkeys let's swing from the trees.
Swing to a branch and pick off some leaves.
Swing to the left, and swing to the right.
Grab a banana and take a big bite.
Cute little monkeys, don't you love to jump?
Whoops you missed that branch and landed on your
rump.
Let's run little monkeys, run fast all around.
And don't you stop 'til you fall on the ground.
REPEAT

(After poem, have kids jump around like monkeys and make
monkey noises.)

Chapter 11

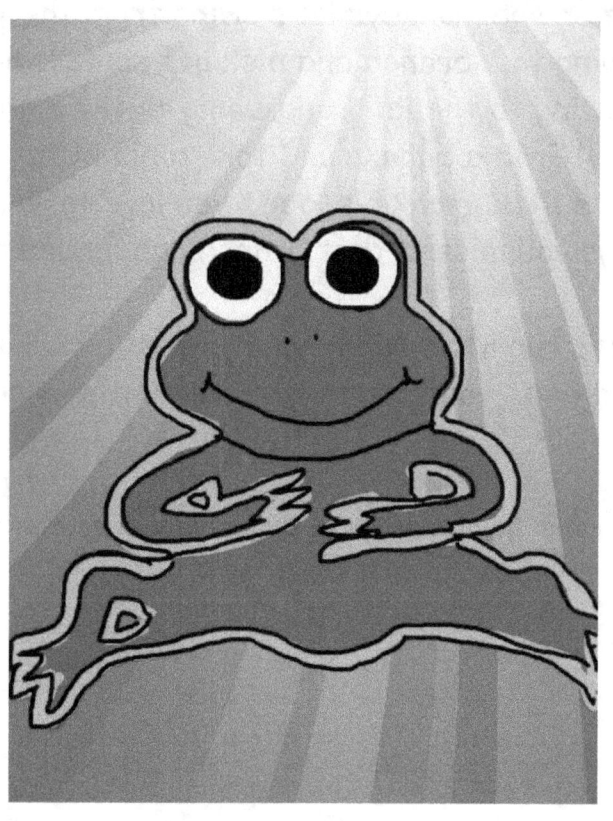

Frog

Hop, hop, hop, hop
Keep on hopping don't you stop.
Hop to the water and jump in the pond.
Hop towards your friends, jump over someone.
Don't hop like a horse.
Don't hop like a dog.
Get on your hopping legs and hop like a frog.
REPEAT

(After poem, have kids play leap frog.)

Chapter 12

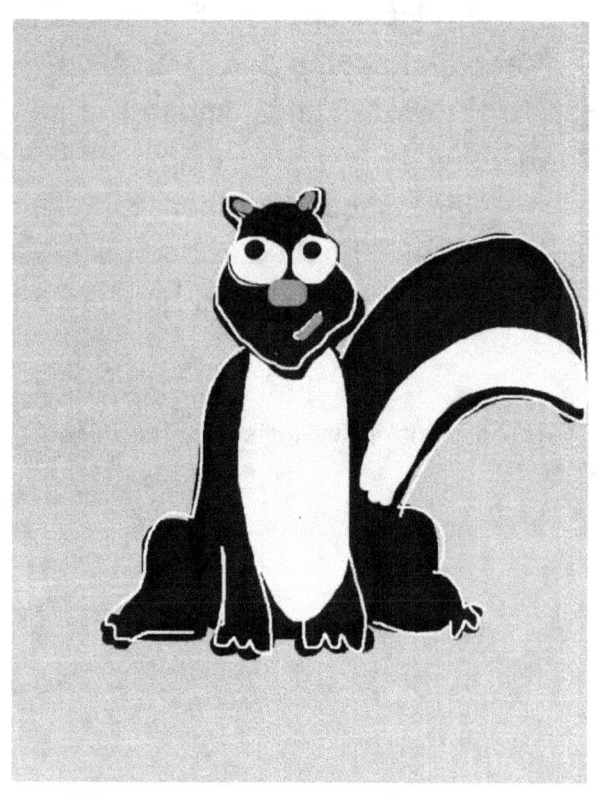

Skunk

Man, oh man, you stinky, stinky skunk,
Stop that smell and shake your trunk.
Don't spray them and don't spray me.
Walk over there and spray that tree.
All skunks smell even all the little ones.
So shake that stinker all over someone.
REPEAT

(After poem, have kids shake their booties in a Congo line.)

Chapter 13

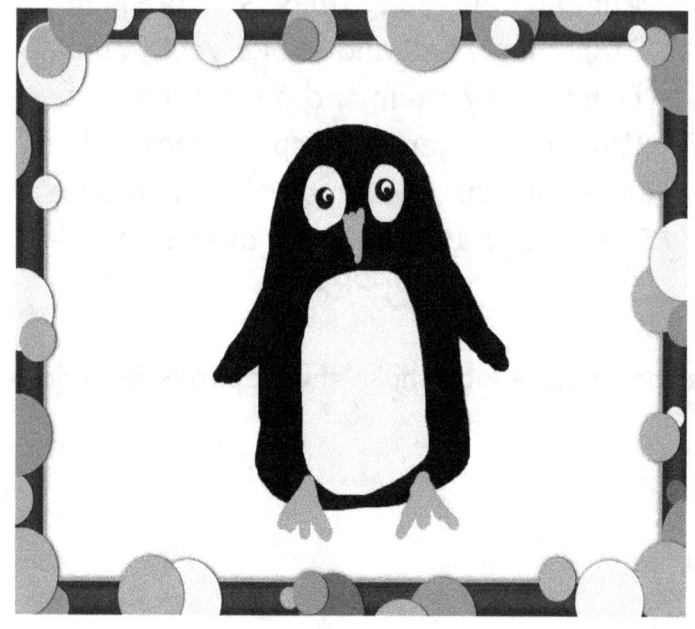

Penguin

To be a penguin you have to waddle round.
And flip those flippers up and down.
Poor little penguin slipping in the snow.
Then fell on the ice and stumped his toe.
Wearing a tux all dressed up.
Pours himself some grape juice in a cup.
Fancy little penguin finds his friend.
Gives her a hug chin to chin.
Sweet little penguins waddle hand in hand.
Flipping their flippers from iceberg to the land.

(After poem, have kids tense and then relax their bodies like
they're freezing and unfreezing. Repeat 3 times.)

Chapter 14

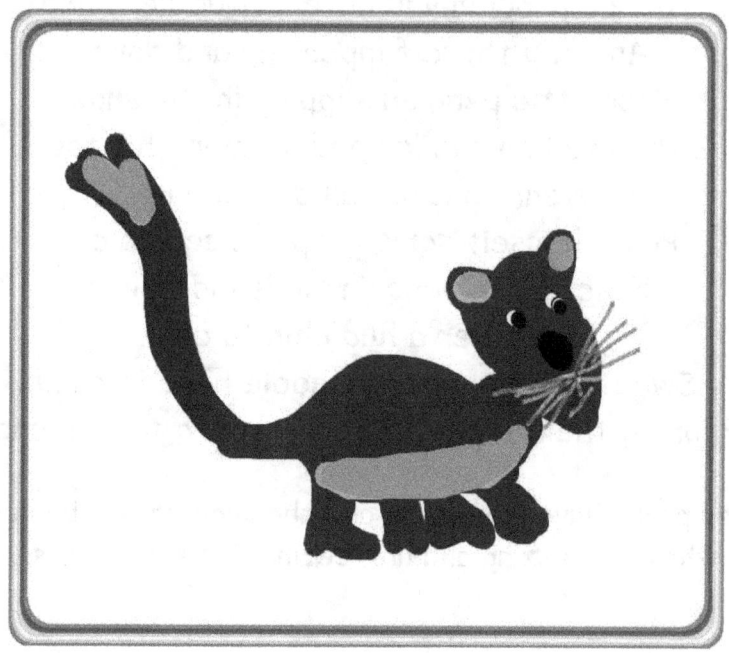

Weasel

Zip, Zap, Zip, Zap
Here comes the weasel, lands on your lap.
He snuggles on down with his cute weasel prance.
Then he stands in front of you and does a weasel dance.
(Dance around crazily)
Zipping and a'Zapping flitting round the room.
Fast little weasel Zoom, Zoom, Zooooom.
REPEAT

(After poem, do a weasel relay race.)

Good Job!

Warm Down!

Chapter 15

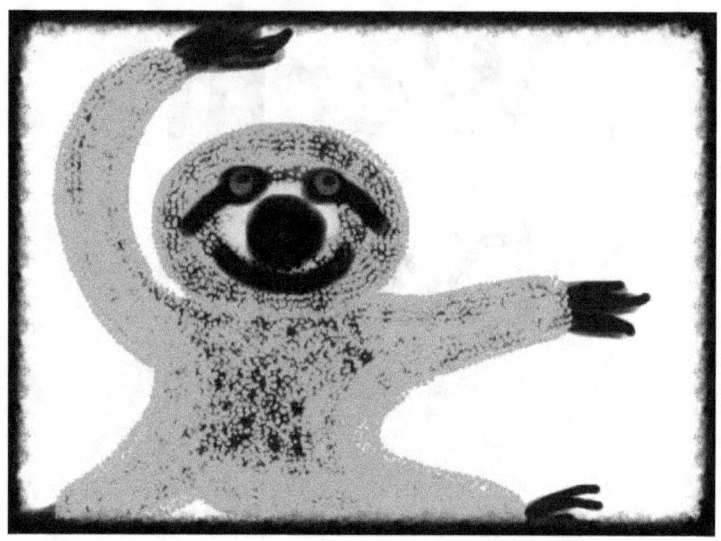

Sloth

The slooooooow sloth hangs from a tree.
Hangs his arms swinging free.
Slow sloth hanging his head.
Moving towards the ground ready for bed.
Sloooow sloth moves very slow.
Moving towards the ground Go, Go, Go.
Bend and stretch right down to your belly.
Now wiggle on the floor like a bowl of jelly.
Now take a deep breath, let it out, count to 3.
And wrap your body round the bottom of a tree.

(After poem, have kids breathe in, count to 3, then breathe
out. Do this 3 times.)

Chapter 16

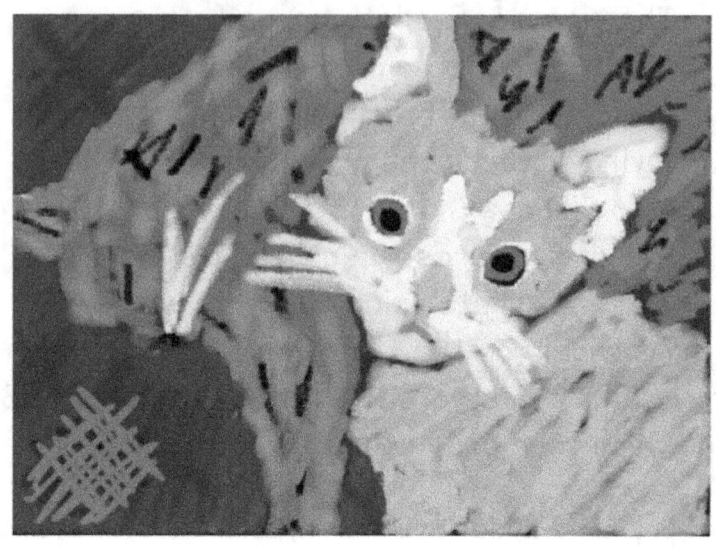

Kitten

Kitten you're so cute when you start to purr.
You seem to really love it when I pet your fur.
You love to sleep, my sweet little baby.
Promise that you'll stay and don't say maybe.
Lie right down on the rug so snug.
Cute little kitten curled up like a bug.

(After poem, give kids a hug!)

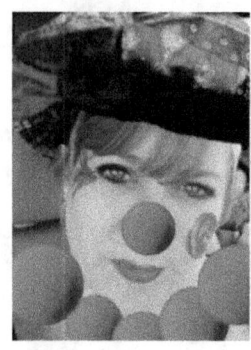 Miss Fanny Pancakes has spent the last ten years entertaining kids. She does everything from puppet shows, to art shows, to exercise shows ...... She has a ton of different voices and sings in her shows as well. Her silliness has won her the prestigious Cranky Hat Award. It is a super secret award, coveted by all circus clowns. Miss Fanny grew up in an invisible circus where her mother was the fake bearded lady and her father the 9 foot tall strongest man. After traveling in the circus until she was twenty she finally settled in a suburb of Los Angeles called Candies End. Candies End allows only people invited there by its residents. A magical town where every day is dress up day and all the houses are made of sugar. Luckily it doesn't rain much. But when it does, a big party is thrown and all the towns' people rebuild their houses.

Look for more books to come from Miss Fanny Pancakes. She has a lot to tell you and looks forward to doing so!

This book was inspired by the last Candy festival in Candies End where too many fatty pounds were found stuck to its residents.

www.ingramcontent.com/pod-product-compliance
Lightning Source LLC
Chambersburg PA
CBHW070842290526
45795CB00002B/957